Foreword

It is with great pleasure that I welcome this report on clinical supervision, which complements the recent publication from my office of Faugier and Butterworth's position paper (1993). It will contribute greatly to the continuing debate on the concept of clinical supervision and play an important part in improving the care which we offer through the development of effective nursing practice.

With the changes which are occurring at present in service provision, the time has never been more opportune for nurses to promote and expand the way in which they contribute to the health service. Seeking innovative ways in which we can respond to patient/client need, while at the same time ensuring that standards of care reach the highest possible levels, is high on my agenda, and I welcome initiatives which offer the opportunity to bring these two principles together.

Exploring, as the report does, the implementation of clinical supervision from a range of different practice settings, highlights many of the issues which nurses will require to take into consideration when introducing it in their own units. The guidelines which are offered here, because they are derived from practice, provide a practical starting point as well as stimulus for discussion.

The enthusiasm and commitment of the practitioners who have contributed is self evident, as is the honesty with which they have shared the challenges this initiative presents. Bringing the practical developments that are taking place in the field together with the theoretical ideas which underpin clinical supervision offers a powerful way of supporting practitioners in developing their work and the quality of patient/client care.

Yvonne Moores
Chief Nursing Officer and Director of Nursing
NHS Management Executive

Introduction

In recent years there has been growing interest in the use of clinical supervision in nursing among both practitioners and managers. Its value as a means not only of developing clinical competence and thus ensuring standards of care for patients but also in supporting staff who often work in difficult and demanding situations has been recognised and there is enthusiasm for both the process and its outcomes. The NHS Management Executive, in 'A Vision for the Future' (1993), recommend that the concept of clinical supervision should be explored and further developed,

'so that it is integral throughout the lifetime of practice, thus enabling practitioners to accept personal responsibility for and be accountable for care and to keep that care under constant review.'

This suggestion has been received with enthusiasm, for reasons that the Management Executive outline:

'Nurses and health visitors require support in the development of their practice One way of providing support is through the process of clinical supervision. Clinical supervision is a term used to describe a formal process of professional support and learning which enables individual practitioners to develop knowledge and competence, assume responsibility for their own practice and enhance consumer protection and the safety of care in complex clinical situations. It is central to the process of learning and to the expansion of the scope of practice and should be seen as a means of encouraging self assessment and analytical and reflective skills.' (NHS Management Executive, 1993)

The value of clinical supervision in nursing has been given additional emphasis in 'The Scope of Professional Practice' (UKCC, 1992a), which gives nurses the freedom to develop their skills in response to patient need. At the same time, there is a clear and fundamental responsibility to ensure that the service that nurses provide for their patients is of the highest possible standard (UKCC, 1992b). Clinical supervision offers a way of enabling staff to develop to meet these demands.

In order to inform continuing work on clinical supervision, this publication documents the experience of five nursing development units where clinical supervision is already in use. These accounts of clinical supervision in practice illustrate the different forms that supervision can take and describe what it is like to give and receive supervision.

The practical experiences of these units form the basis for the guidelines for the introduction of clinical supervision that are summarised opposite. These guidelines are intended as a starting point for those considering the introduction of clinical supervision in their own unit, and provide an agenda for discussion by all those concerned, at every level, in the development of clinical supervision.

Guidelines for the introduction of clinical supervision: **a summary**

For a
discussion
of these
guidelines,
see pages
37 to 42.

1 Before introducing clinical supervision, its purpose should be discussed and clearly defined. This definition should be informed by a theoretical understanding of the role and function of supervision and, equally, by a practical understanding of the circumstances and needs of the unit and its staff.

2 All staff should be involved in the process of planning and introducing a system of clinical supervision.

3 Careful consideration should be given to the qualifications, skills and experience required of supervisors, and to their ability to meet the individual needs of supervisees.

4 All supervisors should be given opportunities to receive training and learn the skills that are needed to provide supervision that is both constructive and supportive. Those who receive supervision should have similar opportunities to learn about their role as supervisees.

5 All supervisors should also receive supervision, in order to monitor and develop the quality of supervision they provide.

6 Supervision should be available to all practitioners, regardless of seniority.

7 The content of supervision should be carefully defined, with boundaries agreed about what is and is not to be dealt with in supervision time. The processes to be used should also be made clear.

8 The relationship between supervisor and supervisee should be formally constituted. Ground rules should be negotiated and agreed.

9 It is essential that clinical supervision is monitored and evaluated. Supervisees and supervisors should play an equal part in these procedures.

10 Individual units need the support of their employing authority to implement and maintain a system of clinical supervision.

The need for clinical supervision

Barbara Vaughan, Director, Nursing Developments Programme, King's Fund Centre

In any role there are good and bad moments and nursing is no different. What is important is that we learn from the experience of our work, building on the strengths and reflecting on what has either been seen as stressful or ineffective, in order that insight can be gained into practice, and clinical competence can be developed.

It was with these thoughts in mind that a recent exploratory study was undertaken at the Royal Liverpool Nursing Development Unit * with the aim of identifying the learning needs of practitioners. Registered nurses were invited to talk about both positive and negative critical incidents which they had experienced in their day-to-day work with a view to finding ways of offering them support.

Making a difference

As is so often the case, it was less easy for these nurses to talk about the things that were good in their practice. Maybe there is a lesson to be learned here, as it is sometimes difficult to find the words to express what is 'expert' in nursing, and it can easily be dismissed as 'nothing special'.

But some of the joys of nursing came through in the stories that were related, and making a difference became an important theme. This nurse, for example, who was working with a patient with cancer:

" . . . I rested my hands lightly on his foot and I gently began to massage. Almost immediately I sensed John beginning to relax. The tension and anxiety disappeared from his face."

Or another nurse who successfuly calmed a patient suffering an acute asthmatic attack and in extreme distress:

". . . I knew it had worked when he fell asleep holding my hand."

What became apparent was that in telling these stories, the nurses involved began to recognise just how skilled they had been. It was not, in these instances, simply a matter of a hand held or stroked but also of getting the timing right and finding a balance between invasion of privacy and offering help. Experiences like these can be recognised by any nurse, regardless of either clinical speciality or experience. Somehow they reflect the feeling of pride which comes when we know that nursing has made a difference.

When it doesn't seem to work

But the impact of nursing is not always apparent and there are times when nurses can be left with feelings of uncertainty, inadequacy and sometimes despair.

"When you are a new staff nurse, you feel so swallowed up and drowning . . ."
"The [extent of the] responsibility of those around me frightened me . . ."

Comments like these were not uncommon in the stories that the nurses told, giving a clear idea of the demands they faced. Patterns could be seen in the stories, and nurses from many different situations were expressing the same demands. The most significant of these were lack of time, limited knowledge on which to base clinical judgement, lack of recognition, and lack of confidence:

ontact:
nn Boon/
are Byrne
oyal Liverpool
ursing
evelopment Unit
Z Link
oyal Liverpool
niversity Hospital
escot Street
iverpool L7 8XP

"You need extra [encouragement and support] . . . to know when you are getting it right and when you are getting it wrong."

Where does all this fit in with clinical supervision? Somehow there had been no structures in the lives of these nurses which gave *them* time. Opportunities were lacking for them to talk about their successes. Equally, mechanisms were lacking which would ensure that worries were picked up and ways found of dealing with them.

For example, in the real world there is no way in which time can be expanded, but help can be given in learning to use time effectively and to prioritise so that some of the guilt and panic are removed and recognition can be given for what *was* achieved. Similarly, recognising a knowledge deficit related to clinical care can mean that learning opportunities are identified, not necessarily through a formal course but by accessing help from experts or time to read.

This team has seen the introduction of clinical supervision as an active way in which they themselves can deal with some of these demands. They know it will not be easy but they reckon it will be worth a try. The decision has been theirs and they are all willing to explore the use of supervision as a means of developing their practice.

As one of them said:

"In nursing we are not going to get away from the bad things in life . . . It's what it is all about, to make those bad things a little bit more bearable for the people involved."

Maybe clinical supervision can make it a little bit more bearable for the nurses too.

Using clinical supervision:
five case studies

Introduction

"Eventually clinical supervision will become part and parcel of everyday nursing, but at the moment we are learning about it all the time."

This section describes how clinical supervision is used in five nursing development units. Each unit has a different approach, although some basic principles are shared. All are in the process of adapting and developing their use of supervision to suit their own particular needs.

The five settings are very different: a community hospital in a rural area, a ward in a long-stay mental health unit, an intensive care unit in a large teaching hospital, an acute mental health unit for adults, and a neighbourhood nursing team in a deprived inner city area. But while the nature and content of the work in these units has influenced, at least to some extent, their implementation and use of supervision, it has not been a major factor.

The information which is presented about the units has been gathered by means of a series of informal interviews with clinical leaders/managers and with those giving and receiving supervision. The aim of these interviews was to collect qualitative information about the experience of implementing and using a supervisory system as well as factual information about the system itself. In the next section (page 37), this information forms the basis for practical guidelines for those considering the implementation of supervision in their own unit.

The five units that are described have not been selected as exemplars. None offer a blue print for others to follow. The purpose in describing their use of supervision is to make their experience available to other units in order to help staff think creatively and critically about their own possible use of a supervisory system.

Case study 1.

Burford Community Hospital, Burford, Oxfordshire

Contact:
Jan Dewing
Lecturer/Practitioner
Burford Community Hospital and Nursing Development Unit
Sheep Street
Burford
Oxon
OX18 4LS

About the unit

This is a community hospital with nine in-patient beds. The hospital operates a twenty-four hour casualty department, a multi-agency day unit, out-patient clinics, and a physiotherapy department. The hospital also organises community support services such as the loan of aids and equipment and carers' groups.

There are twelve whole-time equivalent staff, including the clinical leader/manager, two primary nurses, one full-time associate nurse, six part-time associate nurses, and care assistants, plus a physiotherapist and an occupational therapist. Volunteers work with the staff.

The hospital serves a rural town and its surrounding areas with an overall population of about 20,000.

Why is supervision used in the unit?

The manager/clinical leader of the unit describes the purpose of clinical supervision as to enable nurses to become more effective. She believes strongly in the use of supervision for improving nursing practice and for personal and professional development, and in the educational value of reflective practice. She emphasises, too, that clinical supervision is a necessary and integral part of the culture of the unit and her own style of management.

The present supervisory system

Clinical supervision has been used in this unit for about three and a half years.

The present manager/clinical leader has been in post for two years and until recently she has provided all the supervision herself. One other nurse has now taken on a supervisory role. The manager is a practising nurse educator with considerable experience of giving and receiving supervision.

Individual supervision

Individual supervision is provided for all nursing staff. In future it may also be provided for other qualified staff (for example, the occupational therapist on the unit). The requirement to receive supervision and to keep a reflective diary is included in all nurses' job descriptions.

Supervisions take place every six to eight weeks and last for about an hour. Time-keeping is strict for the sake of other staff:

"We expect all staff to have a commitment to supervision whether or not they are the ones receiving it that day. So if the ward is busy and staff are being asked to hold the fort while someone is having supervision, it helps them to know that it will be for about an hour, or an hour and a half at the most, and that is containable. The time limit is also important for the person receiving supervision because it means they have to make the best use of that time."

Practical arrangements are negotiated and ground rules are discussed and established at the beginning of a supervisory relationship. A contract is made to formalise what is agreed. The most important ground rule is confidentiality - but it is recognised that confidentiality would be broken if a disciplinary matter arose.

Each supervision session is recorded, either on paper or on tape. Initially, notes are taken by the supervisor because in the early stages of supervision, supervisees need to concentrate fully on the process of supervision and may find it difficult to record sessions fully and accurately. Supervisees have the right to challenge the supervisor's recording. As supervisees becomes more used to supervision, they are able to make their own notes. The supervisor and supervisee each keep a copy of the notes. Notes from one session are followed up at the next and progress with set tasks is reviewed. This ensures some continuity and development.

Group supervision

For the last six months, staff have also taken part in group supervision. This has been introduced experimentally, partly in order to explore the possibility of reducing the amount of individual supervision given to more experienced staff by providing group supervision instead. So far, however, both manager and staff (supervisor and supervisees) agree that group supervision has been problematic. Two particular problems have arisen:

● The group included nurses not yet experienced in reflective practice. Other nurses who shared experiences in the group sometimes felt that they were being criticised. The ground rules were therefore re-negotiated. It was agreed that every member of the group had to be committed to supporting colleagues. The supervisor's role within the group was defined as not only to facilitate the overall process but also to attend to the welfare of each member of the group.

● Initially group supervision turned out to be very like individual supervision, but with an audience. This increased people's anxieties about being exposed in the group. To overcome this problem, members of the group were asked to take it in turns to bring in a relevant article (about the practice of therapeutic nursing) for discussion. By this indirect route, it has been possible to achieve some discussion of practice. For the future, the unit is considering using an action learning framework to encourage all members of the group to take an active role in supervision.

The unit will continue to explore the possibility of using group supervision because it seems to offer specific advantages. It is less costly on time, and is potentially team-building:

"What people often talk about in individual supervision is the difficulties they have with their colleagues, and of course the colleagues aren't there. Group supervision is potentially a way of working out new ways of working together."

The content of supervision

Use of reflection

The content of supervision is mostly staff led. Supervisees are encouraged to take control and to bring to the session whatever they wish to discuss. All staff keep private reflective diaries and bring to their supervisions critical incidents which they have recorded in their diaries and reflected on. They use a model of structured reflection to help them do this. In supervision they look at their own handling of the incident: *"What did I do well? What could I have done better?"*

"In supervision, we look at how things could have been done differently. We look at finding new understandings of the process (the 'how'), and then at the skills that are needed to work through the process."

Alternatively, supervisees may choose to focus on an issue which is significant for their practice at that particular time. One nurse, for example, has looked at empathy:

"When I first had supervision, it was mainly about critical incidents, and I got a lot of help and support and new ideas. Then it got to be that I was thinking of the ideas for myself and I didn't need that kind of support so much. So my supervisor suggested that instead of looking at a 'pinpoint' incident, I look at a broader issue and then perhaps narrow down to look at that issue in relation to my work."

The manager also describes the way in which supervisees - and therefore the content and nature of a supervision - progress over time:

"Supervision can begin by being reactive, dealing with things that have happened, things that have gone wrong. It's a 'mopping up' of past experiences, and for the

supervisor, this stage can be hard work for little return. Later it becomes pro-active. People start rehearsing. They say, 'I've got this case conference, I've got this problematic family, this ethical dilemma . . .' And that's when nurses start to become more effective, because they are anticipating problems and asking 'Why am I feeling this way about it? What are the options? What are the consequences? What is the best decision for the patient?'"

The content of supervision is clearly defined as work-related. Personal and private matters are not excluded from supervision but must be relevant to the work experience under discussion. The close relationship between professional and personal qualities is acknowledged:

"In therapeutic nursing, the basis for achieving therapeutic relationships with your colleagues and patients are your personal attributes. So a lot of supervision focuses on critiquing your inner self and bringing forward to the consciousness your motives and feelings."

The gains of supervision and reflection are therefore personal as well as professional because they develop personal knowledge and enable personal growth.

The relationship between managerial and clinical supervision

The manager as supervisor The manager states clearly that, given the culture of this unit, the best person to act as supervisor is the manager herself. The manager describes an approach to management which reflects the nurses' approach to nursing patients.

"In this unit, we are giving patient-centred, holistic care. I lead the staff in the same way. They are all individuals, they all deserve to be treated in certain ways, they are all adults, they have certain rights and also certain responsibilities. My role as manager is to provide a range of services to the staff to enable them to nurse effectively. Part of that service is supervision."

The supervisees point out that one advantage of having ones manager as a supervisor means that it is possible to have informal supervision as needed between more formal sessions.

The manager points out other advantages. For example, nurses who are supervised by their manager can be given instant feedback on their day-to-day practice. The manager also points out that if a purpose of clinical supervision is to change practice, then it is important that the manager should know about it and be involved. However, she acknowledges that nurses may have legitimate reasons for not wanting to be supervised by their manager - for example, because they do not feel comfortable with him or her - although other reasons (such as "wanting the kudos of receiving supervision but not the pain") are not allowable.

The supervisor

The manager stresses that before anyone can act as a supervisor, they first need to have received supervision themselves, and through that, to have learnt reflective practice:

"Once nurses can sustain their own reflection and are self-directing, once they have developed a new level of awareness of themselves as people and of their work, they are then, if they want, ready to start thinking about becoming a supervisor to somebody else."

The manager is conscious of the powerful role that a supervisor plays. She acknowledges that a supervisor comes to possess a large amount of powerful information about the way someone works, and that in the wrong hands a supervision can be highly destructive for the supervisee.

The manager/supervisor receives supervision herself in a group with other senior nurse colleagues from other community hospitals. However, as an experienced, reflective nurse, she feels that she has less need of regular supervision. She points out that conversations with colleagues who are proficient in supervision can become 'mini', spontaneous supervision sessions, and that by supervising others, she continues to learn about herself and her practice.

Qualities of a supervisor

Supervisees describe a supervisor as someone who -
- is completely trustworthy, honest and open
- has good listening and analytical skills
- has greater knowledge of nursing than the supervisee (although peer supervision can also be helpful)
- works in the same environment and the same culture as the supervisee
- is committed to giving supervision.

Supervisees feel that there are advantages to having a supervisor who works within the same unit and therefore knows the patients and situations that they describe. But the manager (in her role as supervisor) comments:

"Sometimes I find it a disadvantage to know the specifics of a patient's case. It means that I have my own ideas and I can be almost waiting to see whether the person I'm supervising says what I want her to say. So although it is quite difficult talking about a case that you don't know, I think if you have a wide enough knowledge and experience of nursing, you understand general principles that you can apply."

The manager describes the most important attribute of a supervisor (and equally, a manager) as sharing the same philosophy as the nurses who are giving care. She also feels that being a supervisor is only possible for a manager with an active, democratic, person-centred style of leadership, who is interested in what the supervisee has to say and who has a good understanding of people. Every supervisor needs his or her own well developed skills in reflection and their own 'internal supervisor':

'The internal supervisor'

"When you are supervising someone, you should be internally supervising yourself at the same time. You need to be very aware of your own motives."

The manager also stresses the supervisor's ability to challenge but also to support, to be non-directive and facilitating, and to be open about the process of supervision.

The relationship between supervisor and supervisee

Supervisees point out that it takes time to build up a good relationship with a supervisor. At the root of that relationship is a commitment on both sides to giving and receiving supervision.

Supervisees say that they feel they have some control of what happens in their supervisions and that as they have become more experienced in receiving supervision, so they have become more able to exercise that control. This means that their relationship with their supervisor does not feel unequal.

Benefits of supervision

Supervisees are enthusiastic about this system and list a number of benefits from their experience of supervision:

- It encourages professional growth. For example, one nurse feels that clinical supervision has enabled her to grow into the role of primary nurse.

- It helps nurses to be more self-assured, more assertive, more confident. They feel supported.

- It helps to broaden thinking by increasing your options.

- It increases a sense of commitment, of professionalism, of status. This is especially helpful for part-time staff.

Supervisees point out that appreciation of these benefits comes slowly. Supervision demands perseverance, but over time, the personal gains become clear.

The supervisor, for her part, is aware of benefits for herself. She feels that as a result of clinical supervision her own managerial role is better understood, and that she has been able to strengthen and improve her relationship with staff.

Case study 2.

Cartmel Ward, Prestwich Hospital, Manchester

Contact:
Nicola Mahood
Senior Nurse
Cartmel Ward
Prestwich Hospital
Bury New Road
Manchester M25 7BL

About the unit

The mental health services of Salford provide a long stay mental health and rehabilitation service among other specialist services. Cartmel Ward caters for up to thirteen highly dependent, elderly men (for whom the average length of stay is thirty-eight years) on the ground floor of the building, and up to twelve semi-independent clients who could not be resettled in the community and who live in four flatlets on the first floor.

The ward is staffed by ten registered mental nurses (RMNs), some with additional specialist qualifications, and nine unqualified staff.

Why is supervision used in the unit?

The impetus to implement supervision in this unit came from a need to be innovative in a service described as 'the Cinderella of the mental health services', and to pay attention to the needs of staff for personal and professional development.

More specifically, clinical supervision was introduced in the unit in order to -

- demonstrate that staff are valued, by investing in them and giving them time for themselves

- provide opportunities for reflection on clinical practice

- improve the quality of client care.

"Often you're not able to talk about your clinical practice unless it's as part of a formal multi-disciplinary case conference or in goal-planning. But even there, you're not given the opportunity to reflect on your skills or discuss them in greater detail. There's not a forum for that. And it seemed that clinical supervision was very much about enhancing your clinical skills and reflecting on your experiences, about being valued, and about developing your career."

13

The present supervisory system

The implementation and development of clinical supervision in this unit has been co-ordinated by a clinical nurse specialist. She now works elsewhere but continues to provide one half-day session a week to the unit and to act as project co-ordinator.

Clinical supervision was introduced in the unit in 1991 and the system has continued to develop in the three years it has been operating. It is now an integral part of the way the unit functions and all job descriptions require that staff receive and, if appropriate, provide clinical supervision. Newly qualified staff receive guidance through preceptorship, whereby they work alongside a named nurse for three to nine months before moving on to clinical supervision.

Individual supervision

Individual clinical supervision is provided for all qualified staff on a regular basis at least once every month. Sessions last for one to one and a half hours and are booked two to three weeks in advance so that the time required can be planned for. Most staff prefer to spend their supervision time away from the ward.

The system is flexible. *"It has to be. Otherwise it would be too easy to cancel."*

Telephone supervision is also available as an informal back-up, so that a nurse can contact his or her supervisor when needed.

Although all qualified staff are expected to receive supervision, the idea of choice and individual responsibility is emphasised:

"Clinical supervision is there primarily to help the supervisee develop. At the end of the day, they're all registered nurses and they're all accountable for their practice. Therefore I think they should be taking responsibility for their supervision as well. I don't think it would work if the manager was behind them saying 'You've got to have supervision'. It's better to motivate people to want it and to be committed to it. And to do that you have to be committed to it yourself . . . and be seen to receive it yourself too."

Each supervision session is recorded on a form developed for the purpose, briefly describing the focus of the session and the perceived benefits to the supervisee. The form is signed by both supervisor and supervisee and is kept by the supervisee. Recording is considered important because without it there would be no means of auditing the system. Apart from the supervisee and his or her supervisor, forms are seen by the supervisee's manager and the clinical supervision project co-ordinator.

Confidentiality

Supervision is regarded as completely confidential but it is recognised that if supervision were to reveal malpractice, this would have to be reported.

"If someone revealed something in supervision that went against the code of professional conduct, then I would have to say to the person, 'Look, I have no alternative but to take that further, but I would prefer you to do it yourself and go and talk to your manager.'"

An evaluation of the present supervisory system has been carried out and benefits were clearly identified. The system will be further developed on the basis of the evaluation results.

The content of supervision

In this unit, clinical supervision is described as a process of identifying skills and deficits, strengths and weaknesses, and working on these in appropriate ways. The main content of supervision is -

- review of, and reflection on, clinical practice
- professional development.

As a guideline, whatever is discussed during supervision should ultimately benefit client care: *"The whole purpose is the benefit to the client."*
     When a supervisor and supervisee first meet, ground rules are discussed and agreed (eg place and frequency of sessions, confidentiality, recording, etc), broad areas to be focused on are identified and a plan made for several months ahead. This plan is adaptable and may be changed or interrupted in order to deal with current concerns. The content of individual supervisions is planned at the beginning of each session, using the record of the previous session to ensure some continuity and cumulative benefit.
     Supervision also provides opportunities to discuss personal feelings and experiences and deal with stress. So, for example, a discussion about the management of a particular incident on the ward may include discussion about the feelings that the incident aroused. In this way, the humanistic, holistic philosophy of the ward in general is reflected in the approach to clinical supervision. Understanding of oneself and others not just as professionals but also as people is considered important:

"As mental health nurses, we're very much encouraged to examine our own beliefs, our values, attitudes, strengths and weaknesses, and to use all our life experiences. The only tools we have are ourselves. We use ourselves in a therapeutic sense. Inherent in this is reflection on ourselves."

The supervisor

When supervision was first introduced in the unit, it was decided that staff should be free to choose their own supervisor. It was hoped that this would help to achieve a relationship in which there was trust and respect. However, experience showed that some standards were needed in order to ensure that supervisors possessed appropriate experience and skills. Criteria have now been set which demand that supervisors -

Criteria for supervisors

- should be able to demonstrate their commitment to updating their theoretical knowledge and skills, and their application of these within the clinical setting, through the completion of a professional and personal profile. The profile should be submitted to an identified panel at twelve monthly intervals to demonstrate the supervisor's continuing commitment to personal development.

- must have a minimum of eighteen months post-registration experience.

- must have participated in a mentorship workshop organised by the local college of nursing.

- must possess a recognised qualification in basic teaching skills or have undertaken a course which incorporates teaching skills.

- must be registered on the rehabilitation service skills register database.

Choice of supervisor Staff have the freedom to choose their own supervisor provided these criteria are met, and it is recognised that there can be a need to change supervisors as staff develop and their needs change. The majority of staff choose supervisors from outside the ward.

All supervisors also receive supervision, from a more experienced but not necessarily more senior person.

Some workshops have been run to provide training for supervisors, and a supervisors' support group is now being set up. A more formal training course would be welcomed. Evaluation of the supervisory system has identified the need for training and development opportunities for supervisors.

Qualities of a supervisor

A supervisor is described as someone who -

- is a good listener

- is supportive, confidence-building and able to give constructive criticism

- facilitates rather than directs

- is able to teach but does not spoon feed

- has good interpersonal skills

- is honest about his or her own limitations.

Supervisees emphasise the importance of feeling able to respect their supervisor in order to be able to accept constructive criticism from him or her. The clinical skills and experience of the supervisor are therefore very important, and while the unit does not stipulate that a supervisor has to be a nurse, no one has ever chosen a supervisor from another discipline.

The relationship between supervisor and supervisee

Clinical supervision is seen as a two-way process involving responsibilities on both sides. The supervisee is not passive but shares the responsibility of making supervision work successfully. A supervisee should be motivated, with a wish to use supervision for personal development; should have some sense of direction; and should be prepared to put thought and effort into the process. Supervision is not 'a time to moan' and although it supports staff, it is not primarily a support system. Its primary purpose is to develop clinical competence.

Although in the mental health services nurses are more used than most to assessing their work and being assessed themselves, a few staff have found supervision threatening. This problem can often be overcome by involving staff and giving choice.

The relationship between managerial and clinical supervision

In this unit, clinical supervision is separate from managerial supervision and serves a different purpose.

Staff may or may not be supervised by their line manager. They are free to choose their supervisor provided certain criteria (see page 15) are met. Their choice is mainly guided by the clinical skills and experience offered by different supervisors. A nurse who wants to develop a particular skill will look for a supervisor who possesses that skill.

At present, the ward manager provides clinical supervision for two nurses whom she also manages. She suggests that they have chosen her as their supervisor because (a) she understands the content of their work and knows their clients, and (b) she has some understanding of their personal concerns. It is likely, and in the manager's view desirable, that these nurses will move on to choose new supervisors outside the ward quite quickly, and this will provide fresh influences as well as a clearer separation between clinical and managerial supervision.

Links between clinical and managerial supervision

Specific links between clinical and managerial supervision are made in two ways:

● Objectives set in individual performance review and staff appraisal may be pursued through clinical supervision. In this way, IPR/appraisal and clinical supervision are co-ordinated and complementary, though separate:

"For example, a staff nurse might have research-based care planning as one of her IPR objectives. So she may ask her clinical supervisor if they can focus on that in supervision. Or during staff appraisal, a nurse may say, 'I feel I need to become more assertive.' And then she could talk about that with her clinical supervisor. It makes a crossover between managerial and clinical supervision. But the supervisor has nothing to do with the IPR or appraisal process, and she is not setting those objectives but helping the supervisee to meet them."

● Each supervisor and supervisee have quarterly meetings with the ward manager in order to deal with any managerial issues which arise in supervision and to check that the direction of the clinical supervision is not at variance with the direction of the unit as a whole.

Benefits of supervision

In this unit, supervision is considered to -

- contribute to improved clinical practice
- have a role in supporting staff
- improve professional development processes
- build staff confidence through positive reinforcement of good practice.

Supervisees list a number of benefits which reflect positive feelings about the challenge that supervision provides:

"I've got a lot of respect for my supervisor and I can take constructive criticism from her. Sometimes you don't like being criticised, even if it's constructive, but sometimes it's something that you need."

"I would say it's definitely improved the quality of my work. We all have some knowledge, but by using someone who's got more expertise than yourself, you can build on what you know."

"The discussion is important because I can examine my own views and use my own knowledge. My supervisor pushes me to examine things more closely, and you realise that you know more than you thought you did."

From the supervisor's point of view, there are personal and also organisational gains:

"It gives me a sense of achievement because I can see the person I supervise has developed a lot and although that's not all down to me, I feel I have helped. It also makes sure that I keep up to date and keeps me on my toes. And it is stimulating and gives me new ideas, which benefit my work and, in the end, the unit."

Contact (in writing):
Jane Simperingham
Eileen Skellern Three Ward
The Maudsley Hospital
Denmark Hill
Camberwell
London
SE5 8BX

About the unit

This is an acute mental health unit for adults with twenty-five beds. The predominant illness dealt with on the ward is acute psychosis, and the average length of stay for patients is four weeks. Staff also provide some follow-up in the community after discharge and the unit has an out-patient caseload of up to ninety patients. There are also up to six patients who attend the unit during the day.

There is an establishment of twenty-five staff, of whom twenty-one are qualified. Nineteen staff are currently in post. The staff work in groups of up to six primary and associate nurses, each group being led by an experienced registered mental nurse.

Why is supervision used in the unit?

Work on this ward is demanding and extremely stressful. The high turnover of patients means that on average there is likely to be at least one admission and one discharge per shift, and at least one episode demanding crisis intervention. In this environment, a system is needed to acknowledge the positive qualities and achievements of staff, review standards of clinical care, and identify individual needs.

The present supervisory system

Clinical supervision is carried out throughout the hospital. It was introduced in this unit in 1990.

All staff receive individual supervision for one hour no less than once a month. Further informal supervision can be arranged in between these

A range of supervisory structures

sessions if staff want and need it. In addition, other supervisory structures are -

- group supervision led by the ward manager for half an hour once a week
- small group meetings for half an hour once a week, led by group leaders
- meetings between the ward manager and group leaders for three hours once a month
- post incident meetings as needed
- informal peer supervision, which is used constantly and as needed.

These structures have been developed gradually in response to need. Post incident meetings, for example, have recently been formalised:

"About six weeks ago, we identified that there was a problem with support. We had a lot of new staff and a lot of people feeling very stressed and we realised we weren't supporting each other. So we began to look at different strategies . . . And while we always did have informal gatherings after an incident, it is now much more structured, more planned, even if it's just for a quick five or ten minutes, just to acknowledge what happened."

Supervision takes place on the ward but in privacy - in the manager's office or staff rooms.

Ground rules are discussed and agreed at the beginning of a supervisory relationship. It is agreed, for example, that sexist or racist comments and insults are not allowed, and that supervision is absolutely confidential, although if any kind of malpractice is revealed, this would have to be reported. This would not be done without the supervisee's knowledge.

It is decided at the start of each supervision session who will take notes. At the end, the supervisor and supervisee review the content of the session and identify and agree specific learning targets, which are then noted down. Notes are kept by the supervisee. These notes are brought back to the next supervision and are used in planning the agenda, so that some continuity is ensured.

Clinical supervision in the unit has been informally evaluated through discussion in the staff group, and the system has been adapted and developed as a result of these discussions. A more formal evaluation is planned.

The content of supervision

Individual supervision

Each individual supervision session follows a similar pattern, beginning with 'time out' in which to relax.

"First we take three minutes to grab a cup of coffee together in the staff room and wind down, because that person has been on shift all morning. Then we go into my office together - as opposed to the person coming in to me."

The supervisor and supervisee then set the agenda for the session together, using a standard format but agreeing priorities for the session and any extra concerns or issues that need to be covered. Areas that are covered are-

- analysis of critical incidents
- review of the supervisee's clinical caseload, looking at how he or she is functioning, at standards of care, and progress with care plans
- the supervisee's supervision of others and development of supervisory skills (if applicable)
- shift management
- personal development and study/training needs.

Goals are set within each area of discussion.

The supervisee may have different concerns or new ideas to bring to the session and the agenda is flexible so that these can be accommodated. In this way, supervision is individual and the content reflects what the individual brings to it.

Personal concerns may also come up in supervision:

"We work in an extremely stressful environment and there is no way our work cannot affect our personal lives. I'm not saying that if you've got personal problems at home then this place is the cause, but it certainly won't help. And rather than someone going off sick, or leaving, because they can't cope with the stress, or coming into work and letting their personal problems affect the standard of care they deliver, I would rather we got those problems out into the open and look at strategies to cope."

The ward manager emphasises that personal and professional lives cannot be separated and that staff support is essential, either informally amongst team members or through external counselling.

Group supervision
In group supervision, the theme for discussion is usually determined by the facilitator for the group. It may focus on a particular patient and the problems relating to his or her care, or it may be a more general theme:

"In our group supervision two weeks ago we were looking at stress and how we weren't supporting each other. The next week there was an obvious improvement in support, and the theme of that group meeting was acknowledgement, and it was a way of saying 'Well done, we're getting there.'"

Individuals may also bring their own concerns to the group. The facilitator will begin by asking those in the group if there is anything they particularly want to discuss.

The supervisor

The manager as supervisor
Until quite recently, clinical supervision has been provided solely by the ward manager/clinical leader, which has proved extremely demanding. It has taken some time for other members of staff to accept the

responsibility of providing supervision, or to accept that supervision can be provided by other staff as well as the manager. However, some primary nurses are now taking on a supervisory role.

Primary nurses who provide supervision also receive it, as does the ward manager:

"I certainly welcome formal supervision for myself. In addition, I've developed my own informal system of peer supervision externally. I think it is extremely important to sit back, take stock, check direction and review the quality of the service I'm delivering."

It is emphasised that at least one year's experience of receiving supervision is needed in order to develop the skills that are needed to supervise others. The supervisor is seen as fulfilling an extremely responsible key role, and the quality of supervision as dependent on the skills of the supervisor.

No particular qualifications or criteria are set to determine who can provide supervision but in general the supervisor's skills and competence are seen as extremely important. Primary nurses who have now begun to provide supervision were judged, and judged themselves, to be ready and able to do so on the basis of their clinical experience, their experience of supervision and their known skills, as well as their personal qualities.

Qualities of a supervisor

The manager describes a supervisor as a teacher and facilitator with a good knowledge base, and as someone who -

- has good teaching and motivational skills
- is a skilled and experienced practitioner
- has basic common sense
- can be confrontational when necessary
- gives positive feedback
- is objective
- is flexible, allowing the supervisee to bring his or her own agenda to supervision.

"A supervisor also needs to take supervision seriously enough to prepare for it adequately in advance. It's no good just giving back to the supervisee what has happened in the last two days. A supervisor needs to develop good observational skills and exercise them all the time."

Staff who receive supervision mention qualities of a rather different kind. They describe a supervisor as someone who is compassionate, wise, kind, honest, knowledgeable, available and approachable.

The relationship between supervisor and supervisee

Both supervisors and supervisees emphasise the need for trust and respect in their relationship. Supervisees feel strongly that they could not respect or relate to a supervisor who was not also a nurse. It is also seen as particularly important that clinical supervision is provided by someone with understanding of, and practical involvement in, the ward's work. The manager's acceptability as a supervisor may be due to the fact that she is

"not someone who sits in an office all day but is out on the shop floor and prepared to get her hands dirty."

Supervisees feel that a close working relationship between them and their supervisor is helpful because of their possible need to bring personal matters to supervision.

"The nature of this job is such that if you're having personal difficulties, like a relationship break-up or a bereavement, then you need to work it through. A supervisor isn't a counsellor, but he or she has the skills to help you reflect on your practice."

The relationship between managerial and clinical supervision

Clinical supervision was initially introduced by the ward manager as an integral part of her approach to management. At that time it was not called clinical supervision, although the fundamental principles were apparent. Now, clinical and managerial supervision remain closely linked. The manager feels that providing clinical supervision for her staff enables her to care for their welfare, gauge their morale and understand their needs, as well as to help them to develop their clinical practice. She feels that this understanding is essential if she is to manage the ward effectively.

It is felt that clinical supervision necessarily reflects (and to some extent helps to cultivate) the ward philosophy. This argues in favour of a close relationship between clinical and managerial supervision, since a supervisor from outside the ward may not share the same philosophy:

"I feel it is important that we develop cohesion and agree on standards of care within the unit. Clinical supervision helps us do that."

Benefits of supervision

Staff feel that supervision -

- provides acknowledgement of their stress and heavy workload

- provides guidance which enables them to develop and progress

- identifies skills that they either possess or need

- is motivational

- is an opportunity to vent feelings connected with work, such as anger, indignation, or revulsion
- provides perspective, helping them to take a more reasonable and objective view of their work
- enables them to support each other in a more organised way.

Supervision is seen as very positive. Staff describe a 'culture of supervision' which they feel now exists on the ward and which enables them to be more constructive.

"It's easy on a ward like this, or on any ward, to just sit back and whinge about things and I think what supervision certainly does for me is encourage me to actually tackle these things I'm whinging about and to try and change things. It gives me that motivation and guidance."

"I think I have certainly changed and progressed an awful lot since I've been here and I don't think I could have done that without supervision. It identifies the areas that I need to work on, the skills I've got and the skills I need to develop, the knowledge that I need to develop. And it gives me the encouragement and support to really go for things."

Case study 4.

Intensive Care Unit, Chelsea and Westminster
Hospital, London

Contact:
Kim Manley
Clinical Nurse Specialist
Intensive Care/Nursing Development Unit
Chelsea and Westminster Hospital
369 Fulham Road
London
SW10 9NH

About the unit

This is a six-bed general intensive care unit. Patients come to the unit
from the accident and emergency department, or post surgery, or
because they have become critically ill elsewhere in the hospital. Patients
are also transferred from other hospitals.

There are currently thirty-five staff in post and the unit is recruiting to
raise staff numbers to forty-two because of expanding services. The staff
as a whole is experienced and well qualified. At least two thirds have
additional qualifications in intensive care and a third are graduates or
undergraduates in nursing.

The staff work in six teams, each team having responsibility for one
patient. Each team has a similar skill mix and is led by a team co-
ordinator. There are six nurses to a team, one of whom acts as a primary
nurse and the others as associates within the team. A different primary
nurse is designated for each new patient.

The unit aims to provide a personalised service, which is family centred
and provides continuity of care.

Why is supervision used in the unit?

The unit aims, through a system of supervised reflective practice, *"to
improve our personal knowledge and our effectiveness as nurses."*

*"We needed to develop that knowledge because we were practising primary nursing.
To develop a therapeutic relationship with patients one has to know oneself and be
able to use oneself therapeutically."*

The present supervisory system

Note: In this unit, clinical supervision (using supervised reflective practice) and managerial supervision (using systems of staff orientation, individual performance review and preceptorship) run in parallel but complement each other. Although both systems are described within the unit as clinical supervision because both, in different ways, are seen to be about staff development and clinical practice, the following account focuses on the unit's use of supervised reflective practice.

Supervised reflective practice

A clinical nurse specialist working in the unit as an advanced practitioner and educator (among other roles) has helped to develop a system of supervised reflective practice. The system is still in its early stages. The unit has also bought in expert help from an outside supervisor as it was felt that the necessary supervisory skills were not available within the unit and staff needed to develop practical experience in being reflective and supervising others.

Group supervision

As a first stage in this learning process, group supervision was initiated for team co-ordinators a year ago. The team co-ordinators met for two hours every two weeks with the clinical nurse specialist and an outside supervisor. These meetings took place mainly in the nurses' own time, and the unit points out the high level of commitment that was therefore required.

Group supervision was chosen rather than individual supervision for pragmatic reasons (to do with staff time) and because it speeded up both the learning process and the implementation of the supervisory system.

Group supervisions were initially designed to help participants become reflective practitioners. Everyone in the group brought to each supervision an experience from their own practice. They wrote up their experiences using a model of structured reflection (Johns, 1994). At each session, one or two nurses shared their experience with the group and were supervised within the group to reflect more deeply on it.

The writing up of the experience is seen as important:

"We agreed that before we brought an experience to the group we had to have reflected on it and internalised it. Writing it down was part of that, because you can go over something in your head but it actually does help to write it down."

Initially, supervision was provided solely by the outside supervisor. Later, in order to develop group members' own supervisory skills, supervision was shared and everyone within the group was given the opportunity to act as supervisor.

Group supervisions for team co-ordinators continue to take place but are now held once a month and have a different purpose, which is to reflect on the supervision that team co-ordinators now provide for colleagues.

Individual supervision

Individual supervision by team co-ordinators has begun in the last two months. Each team co-ordinator supervises one volunteer from within his or her own team.

"Staff currently volunteer for individual supervision because we are introducing change according to our beliefs - that is, in a participative way. We recognise this demands a high level of commitment. However, there is an expectation in the unit that staff will be reflective, and we are beginning to introduce this idea when recruiting new staff."

Individual supervisions take place ideally every three weeks and use the same model of supervised reflective practice. Supervisees record in a personal journal any experiences that they wish to reflect upon. These journals are confidential: they are not shared with supervisors. The supervisee chooses an experience from his or her journal to bring to supervision, and presents it in writing.

Ground rules are formally agreed and recorded on paper at the beginning of a supervisory relationship.

The supervisor takes notes during the supervision session and these are written up afterwards and validated by the supervisee at the next meeting.

"We are all trying to develop good note-taking skills, because it is certainly a very difficult thing to do, especially because you have to take notes and supervise at the same time. The main thing is to capture the spirit of what is said, and we use the supervisee's own words as much as possible. It helps that supervisees bring their experiences already written up."

Written experiences are collected in a folder and every six months supervisees use these documents and their personal journals to carry out a reflective review of their experiences during that time. This review is also written up and shared with the supervisor.

"The aim is to look at how reflective practice has helped them, what themes are emerging, and how they want to develop in the future. This can change the direction of supervision. They may, for example, find that a previously unidentified theme is surfacing and in the next six months they may choose to address this."

The content of supervision

The purpose of supervision is to help nurses become more effective in their work, so the content of supervision is always work-related.

The specific content is largely determined by the supervisees. Both in group and individual supervision, supervisees bring to each session an experience on which they have reflected and which they have chosen to discuss. In the case of the team co-ordinators, experiences that are brought to supervision tend to focus more on managerial issues than on patient care and, latterly, on their provision of supervision to others.

In group supervision, team co-ordinators found that they could readily identify with the situations and experiences brought to supervision by their colleagues:

"It was very much, 'Oh, I've been there!'"

The relationship between managerial and clinical supervision

Managerial and clinical supervision are separated (as described on page 26) but there is a clear relationship, or crossover, between the two. Individual performance review (IPR) is used to set objectives, and supervised reflective practice can be chosen to evaluate progress in meeting those objectives.

Comple-mentary roles of manager and supervisor

Team co-ordinators who combine the roles of manager and supervisor acknowledge the potential tension in this combination but also feel that the roles can be complementary.

"I was doing an IPR with a senior member of my team yesterday. She outlined her strengths and then went on to look at her areas for development, and it seemed clear to me that reflective practice would be very useful, both in relation to her areas for development in order to give her positive feedback, and to help her achieve her objectives.

"So I felt, yes, it's possible to undertake both roles, and they may complement each other. But there has to be respect and trust within that relationship. Otherwise staff will not be willing to share their weaknesses and things they feel are wrong about their practice with me as their manager, since I'm the person they'll be applying to for promotion and references."

The relationship between management and supervision is, in any case, seen as something that has always existed.

"As team leaders we have always had some kind of responsibility to help and 'supervise' members of our team as well as to manage them. Supervised reflective practice has made that more explicit, concrete and formal."

The supervisor

Staff on this unit have only recently taken on supervisory roles. Prior to this, they have received group supervision for one year and through that process they have learnt to be reflective. They have also learnt and practised supervisory skills and continue to receive supervision to enable them to reflect on their provision of supervision. Continuing supervision for supervisors is considered important.

It is seen as essential that supervisors are committed to developing and supporting others, and have an overall commitment to the development of nursing practice.

Qualities of a supervisor

The clinical nurse specialist on this unit identifies the qualities of a supervisor as -

- an expert facilitator
- someone who has extensive knowledge of nursing, in order to be able to help supervisees make sense of their experiences, but someone who recognises their own limitations. When necessary, a supervisor should be able to direct a supervisee to others with different knowledge and expertise.

It is helpful if the supervisor shares the supervisee's speciality, but this is not essential.

Supervisors challenge supervisees but also support them, creating an environment which is summarised as 'high challenge and high support'.

"For example, you might bring to the supervisee's attention contradictions in what they're saying. That's one way of providing high challenge. You're saying, 'Right. Your philosophy says this, and you're doing this.' But you're also saying, 'Look, it's tough in the real world. Very tough.' That's the support. The supervisor has to be very skilled and sensitive to do this. It is also evaluated at the end of the session, so the supervisor then asks the supervisee how much challenge and how much support they have experienced."

Staff also mention the importance of the supervisor's understanding. As experienced and knowledgeable practitioners, supervisors may feel, as the clinical nurse specialist on the unit put it, that *"it's a long time since I've done anything I feel unsure about."* But remembering what it is like to feel less certain about ones practice and to experience stress as a result of uncertainty or inexperience is an important quality in a supervisor.

The relationship between supervisor and supervisee

Use of an external supervisor

Group supervision for team co-ordinators has to date been facilitated by an expert, outside supervisor. Although the nurses who have been receiving group supervision feel completely assured of the supervisor's credentials and emphasise the benefits of receiving supervision from an experienced supervisor with a very extensive knowledge base, nonetheless they also admit to some uncomfortable feelings. These arose not just from the experience of having their own practice challenged but also from the fact that the supervisor was not a practitioner on the unit and therefore had not experienced the same stresses or pressures as supervisees.

In individual supervision (which is still at an early stage of development on the unit), it is felt to be essential that supervisees can respect and trust their supervisors, and choice plays a part in establishing a trusting relationship. Supervisors are in effect chosen by supervisees because staff volunteer for supervision.

Benefits of supervision

Team co-ordinators on the unit feel that nurses have valuable knowledge and expertise to offer but need to learn how to use their professional skills more effectively. Supervision helps them do this.

"Many of the issues faced by team co-ordinators are to do with the way the multidisciplinary team functions. Nurses need to become more assertive in putting forward their perspective. Supervision and reflective practice have enabled them to acknowledge and look at conflicts within the multidisciplinary team."

Team co-ordinators who have taken part in group supervision also list other benefits of supervised reflective practice, about which they feel very positive. For them, group supervision has -

- improved relationships between team co-ordinators and team members

- helped them to examine their own practice in a thoughtful and critical way, but also to have confidence in their own skills and, sometimes, in their intuitive knowledge

- increased their awareness of problems in their own practice or in the service that is given to patients and families, and encouraged them to tackle those problems

- increased a sense of community among group members through new awareness of shared problems

- increased personal and professional self-awareness

- taught that challenge can be a good thing

- provided positive feedback - something that nurses frequently lack.

Apart from these gains for themselves, their teams and the unit, staff describe the ultimate purpose of supervised reflective practice as promoting better quality of care for patients:

"Reflective practice enables nurses to develop. Development is emancipating, and the results of that emancipation can be seen in the quality of patient care."

Case study 5.

Stepney Neighbourhood Nursing Team,
Steels Lane Health Centre, London

Contact:
Julia James
Clinical Leader (Acting)
Steels Lane Health Centre
384 Commercial Road
London
E1 0LR

Note: This unit does not use the term 'clinical supervision' to describe the system of supervision, development and support that is offered to staff. Members of the team who receive 'supervision' are strongly opposed to the term. They emphasise their autonomy as qualified professionals with particular areas of practice and expertise. For them, the term 'supervision' threatens this autonomy, as the manager explains:

"Although community nurses are more familiar than most nurses with supervision as a concept because of their proximity to social work, it still feels uncomfortable and threatening to have someone supervise you. Most community nurses have picked this sphere of nursing to get away from control and lack of autonomy over their own practice."

Nevertheless, both the manager and members of the team are aware of the points of contact between their own system and clinical supervision. The word 'supervision' is used (though sparingly) in this account to illustrate this.

About the unit

The Stepney Neighbourhood Nursing Team was formed in 1990. It is based in two health centres and a clinic, all within a one-mile radius. The team serves a population of about 27,000 people in an inner city area which is socially and economically deprived, with poor housing and high levels of unemployment, family breakdown and domestic violence. The population is multi-ethnic, including groups who do not speak English, and suffers the health and social problems that spring directly from poverty.

There are forty-five members of staff in the present multi-disciplinary team. Most are district nurses, health visitors and school nurses. Others are specialist community nurses and support workers. Staff range from very inexperienced to very experienced and highly qualified. The team is managed by a community nurse, who is also the clinical leader.

Why is supervision used in the unit?

'Active management'

When the neighbourhood nursing team was formed in 1990, the manager introduced a system of individual meetings with staff initially in order to get to know them, learn about their jobs (since she did not share all their specialties), and establish good working relationships. There were then twenty-five staff in the team.

"I called it 'active management', because I was coming into a service that had been traditionally under-managed. People had been left to their own devices, there was no training, career development or planning with staff in any formal way. Individual meetings with staff did not happen."

This style of management is now seen as a vital way of building and maintaining good relationships in the team and of working together creatively. The manager believes *"that it is investment in staff that produces developments in practice."*

The present supervisory system

Individual meetings

The manager meets individually with each member of staff no less than once every eight weeks for about forty-five minutes to an hour.

"Every practitioner has a set of objectives that they develop with me and we agree. Their whole work should be described within these objectives. We use our regular meetings as a process of continual review rather than having formal appraisal on, say, an annual basis."

The supervisor and supervisee usually take turns to write the minutes of the meeting and these are typed up. Apart from the typist, the minutes are only seen by the two people involved and are confidential, with the agreed exception of disciplinary matters. Occasionally, the content of a session may be shared with other team members if it seems of interest, provided this is agreed by the supervisor and supervisee.

The agenda for each meeting is set on the basis of the minutes of the last, with new items added. Both the manager and the nurse come to each meeting with new items to discuss.

Communication and team-building strategies

In addition to these individual meetings with staff, a number of strategies are used in the unit to ensure good communication, team-building and high standards of care. These include business meetings with particular groups of staff (such as health visitors or school nurses); monthly team meetings; and mentorship within 'mini-teams' of approximately eight people. Within these mini-teams, more experienced staff act as mentors for less experienced team members and meet with them to talk about individual and team objectives. In district nursing in particular, this is starting to result in the devolution of supervision from the manager to the G-grade qualified district nurses.

Use of a child protection adviser

Staff also have access to a child protection adviser - an experienced fieldworker who provides supervision, advice and support to staff specifically in relation to child protection and, occasionally, some other especially difficult areas of their work. The adviser is available to staff at all times and sees individuals regularly every three to six months to formally review their child protection work.

Informal peer supervision is also encouraged in the unit. The manager uses her knowledge of her team to link staff who can offer each other relevant skills and experience. The manager herself keeps an 'open door' for all her staff. In these ways, the clinical expertise available within the unit is used to the full.

The content of supervision

The purpose of the manager's individual meetings with staff is to -

- set objectives for practice for each individual

- help staff with the management of their work load and with associated stress

- help staff accommodate plans for changing the way they or their teams work

- discuss each individual's professional development, including training needs.

Staff feel it is possible to take anything they wish to discuss to their meetings with their manager, including personal concerns, although they feel that on the whole, personal matters are best talked about elsewhere. Discussion usually covers their recent progress at work, any difficulties they are encountering, and their objectives and professional development. They prefer to describe what they receive as advice, support and professional guidance, rather than 'supervision'.

The relationship between managerial and clinical supervision

In this unit, clinical and managerial supervision are wholly integrated. Supervision is seen as a way of managing, but as achieving more:

"It's more than simply managing, more than making sure that staff are doing the job they're paid to do. It's about helping people to grow, helping people to stay healthy, and maintaining the quality of services. And it means that if staff have got problems,

either personal or about their case work, they know me well enough and trust me enough to bring those problems to me."

The manager is aware that this aspect of her work as an operational manager is the part which is least recognised and, without organisational support, the part which most risks being 'squeezed'.

Only supervision in the area of child protection is separated from management because of the large workload this entails. In this area, supervision is provided by a child protection adviser (see above) who has received special training not only in child protection but also in the provision of supervision itself. Her role is to support practitioners, help them develop and maintain high standards of practice, and assess training needs. This scheme is highly valued by both managers and practitioners and is felt to be a model that could be easily transferred elsewhere.

The supervisor

Almost all supervision is undertaken by the manager. She estimates that this uses about thirty hours of her time per month, including time for administrative back-up work. In her view, it is time well spent:

"My job is to facilitate the development of practitioners so that they develop practice, and by developing their practice, they provide better services to clients. If that is my job, as I believe it is, then I have no choice. It is, quite simply, labour-intensive, getting the best out of people."

The manager herself does not receive supervision or management of a similar kind, although she receives support from her professional organisation. Nonetheless, she feels the lack of other people who perceive management in the same way that she does:

"I would love to have someone do for me what I do for my team."

Qualities of a supervisor

The manager suggests that she is using very similar skills with staff as she uses with clients, including facilitation and negotiation skills, working in partnership, being open. She also emphasises the importance of helping staff deal with stress, providing support for them to achieve more, and giving positive feedback.

In the view of the staff, a manager who uses this style of management must be -

- professionally up-to-date
- able to respect the autonomy and professionalism of staff
- trustworthy
- non-judgemental
- not frightened of change

- open and communicative
- a good, active listener.

The relationship between supervisor and supervisee

There is a very high degree of trust between the manager and members of the team. The manager points out that it takes time to build this trusting relationship, *"and the NHS isn't good at things that take a long time to produce dividends."* Team members, for their part, attribute their positive relationship with their manager to mutual professional respect and a 'hands on' style of management:

"She respects our clinical expertise and professionalism and doesn't impose. She lets you take control of your case load. On the other hand, she doesn't just wait vaguely around in the background. She does like to know what's going on."

Staff are clearly not dependent on the manager for support. They have found their own sources of support and feel this is important for the manager's sake as well as their own:

"There isn't time to go to your manager about everything and there isn't the need either. You build up your own support networks. If you unloaded everything on to your manager, she wouldn't be able to do her job."

Benefits of supervision

Team members are clear that they benefit from the style of management used in this unit. They say that it gives them individual recognition, a sense of their own worth, and a sense of being valued as a team member. They point to the benefits of discussing their case work and identifying their training needs.

"I would find it threatening if she tried to instruct me on how to manage a particular case but she never has. She says, 'Well, these are your options. You could do it that way or this way. What do you think?' And she hands it back to you."

The manager suggests that benefits for her team are:

● They have a manager who understands what they are doing and why, and who is helping them to match the hours available and their skills with the job that is to be done.

● They receive help in building their professional portfolio, identifying training needs, and finding ways to meet those needs.

"Particularly in a recession, people don't have the same opportunities to change jobs. So they have got to have a career plan. They may be stuck in jobs they don't necessarily want to stay in, and they have got to keep growing in that job. It is essential for them and for the service they provide that they continue to get something out of their work."

● The team itself is strengthened.

There are also clear benefits for clients:

"Clients benefit from an environment in which new things can be tried and risks can be taken, and services changed and made responsive to their needs. This cannot be achieved if people are feeling demoralised and overburdened, and it is my job to take away that stress."

Finally, there are benefits for the manager herself:

"I get to know my team really well. I get a lot of support from them. I don't have this 'I'm the manager, they're the staff' separation. I don't feel completely isolated from them as my peer group. It keeps me close to practice, close to their clients. I see myself as part of the team."

Introducing clinical supervision:
practical guidelines

These guidelines are based on the practical experience of the five nursing development units described in the previous section. They offer a general framework for the introduction of clinical supervision. They also highlight some of the main issues which emerged from interviews in the nursing development units.

> **Before introducing clinical supervision, its purpose should be discussed and clearly defined. This definition should be informed by a theoretical understanding of the role and function of supervision and, equally, by a practical understanding of the circumstances and needs of the unit and its staff.**

Clinical supervision may be used to meet the needs of staff for professional development, support and management. The corresponding functions of supervision are described by Proctor (1986) as -
- formative (the educative process of developing skills)
- restorative (supportive help for professionals working constantly with distress and stress)
- normative (the managerial and quality control aspects of professional practice).

However, clinical supervision can be used in a variety of ways. Different units may choose to emphasise different functions and/or exclude others. For example -
- clinical supervision may be used for all three purposes of development, support and management. In this case, supervision will be provided by the manager or line manager. There will be clear links with individual performance review (IPR).
Or
- clinical supervision may be separated from management and staff support and used solely in its formative role. In this case, supervisors can be chosen for the specific experience, expertise and skills that they offer. Systems for managerial supervision and for staff support will exist alongside, and links will need to be made between clinical and managerial supervision, including IPR.

These are just two alternatives and many other systems are possible.

In order to devise a system that is suited to their circumstances and needs, each unit first needs to clarify and agree the role and purpose of clinical supervision in the light of their existing structures, available resources and, most important, the needs of the unit and its staff.

2 **All staff should be involved in the process of planning and introducing a system of clinical supervision.**

Clinical supervision demands a high level of commitment from staff at all levels. This commitment is both practical and philosophical. Practically, there has to be a willingness to expend time and effort; philosophically, there has to be a belief in the effectiveness and benefits of a supervisory system. All staff must be prepared to look critically at the quality of their own practice.

Because of the demands that supervision places upon staff individually and as a team, it is vital that staff are involved in planning for the introduction of clinical supervision, and subsequently in the process of implementation.

It may be helpful for staff -

- to be informed about and have the opportunity to discuss what clinical supervision is and what it offers to them and to the unit
- to discuss and clarify the need for supervision in relation to their own everyday practice and their personal and professional development
- to discuss the potential benefits for the unit as a whole in terms of team building and the quality of client care
- to be given the opportunity to express doubts and anxieties and ask questions
- to define, agree and jointly own aims for the use of supervision in the unit.

3 **Careful consideration should be given to the qualifications, skills and experience required of supervisors, and to their ability to meet the individual needs of supervisees.**

Each unit needs to consider carefully who can provide clinical supervision most appropriately and effectively. It is essential that all those who fulfil a supervisory role possess the qualifications, skills and experience that the unit's system of supervision requires, and at an individual level, that they are able to meet the needs of supervisees.

The following questions, among others, may need to be debated:

• Should each member of staff be able to choose his or her supervisor? What guidance should be given, and what constraints should there be?

• Should supervisors be required to fulfil certain agreed criteria, in order to ensure that they possess appropriate experience, qualifications and skills? If so, what criteria?

• What personal qualities should a supervisor ideally possess? Should personal qualities be taken into account in deciding who should supervise, and if so, how?

• How much time will the supervisor need to give to the provision of supervision. How can that time be made available?

• How many supervisees can any one supervisor be expected to supervise effectively?

• Is it important that the supervisor should have day-to-day contact with a supervisee and be acquainted with his or her work, colleagues and clients? Or could this be a disadvantage?

• Could a supervisor face conflicting interests or responsibilities in providing supervision for practitioners within his or her own team?

In units where managerial and clinical supervision are combined, supervision will be provided by the manager of the unit and/or line managers. However, there is still a need to consider what the manager as supervisor can and cannot offer, since a manager may not possess all the skills that are needed or may not be the most appropriate supervisor in certain circumstances. It may, for example, be more appropriate for a practitioner who is under particular stress to be supported by a person other than his or her manager. It is important to identify unmet needs and ensure these needs are met in other ways.

Particularly in the early developmental stages of implementing supervision, difficulties in finding sufficient and appropriate supervisors for staff may be overcome in a number of different ways. Some options to consider are:

• group supervision

• the use of supervisors outside the unit (which may be particularly appropriate for managers and clinical leaders)

• reciprocal arrangements with other units

• provision of resources for senior staff to learn supervisory skills.

---

4 **All supervisors should be given opportunities to receive training and learn the skills that are needed to provide supervision that is both constructive and supportive. Those who receive supervision should have similar opportunities to learn about their role as supervisees.**

All supervisors need to learn (or to have learnt) basic skills and should also have opportunities to build on those skills, and to review and evaluate their provision of supervision at regular intervals.

Since the supervisory role is potentially an extremely powerful one, it is also essential that supervisors are aware of their responsibilities and can work within proper constraints. This too is a matter for training and not merely of personal integrity.

In the absence of any formal training from an appropriate national body, units currently have to devise their own ways of ensuring that supervisors have the skills they need to supervise well. These may include:

• providing workshops and training days

• facilitating discussion and learning in groups

• providing continuing supervision for supervisors (see below)

• using other courses and qualifications with relevant components
eg management, teaching or counselling

• enabling new and inexperienced supervisors to learn from those who are experienced, through individual or group supervision

• requiring practitioners to receive supervision for an agreed minimum period before becoming supervisors.

Alongside such initiatives, there remains a pressing need for formal training in supervisory skills. At a local level, it may be possible to negotiate with a local college of further or higher education to provide an appropriate training module. Relevant training expertise may also be available from professionals in other disciplines.

It is also helpful for those who receive supervision to have similar opportunities to learn about their own role as supervisees, and about how they can make best and maximum use of supervision. The supervisory relationship can be mutually beneficial, and in order to enhance that relationship, and to ensure that the supervisee is fully aware of the processes at work in supervision and is able to benefit fully from them, units should consider ways of enabling supervisees to learn about, analyse and discuss the experience of receiving supervision.

5 **All supervisors should also receive supervision, in order to monitor and develop the quality of supervision they provide.**

Providing supervision is demanding and difficult, both personally and professionally, and those who provide supervision should therefore be entitled to receive similar support. This should help to ensure that they supervise well, that they continue to develop their supervisory skills, and that they have the personal support they need to deal with any difficulties.

Supervision for supervisors is also essential in order to monitor the service they provide. It is, or should be, a safeguard for both supervisor and supervisee.

6 **Supervision should be available to all practitioners, regardless of seniority.**

The UKCC (1993) suggest that 'practitioners have no end point in their need to maintain and develop standards of practice.' Supervision, which is often seen as a provision for less experienced practitioners, still plays an important role in professional development for senior staff, but with a different focus and content. For example, a manager who identifies a need to develop his or her skills in financial management, team-building, strategic planning or other similar areas, should be able to use supervision to do so.

In order to find appropriate supervisors, senior staff are likely to have to look outside their own unit, and may sometimes find it useful to work with colleagues from other disciplines. Such arrangements should be facilitated by the employing authority.

Ideally, the giving and receiving of clinical supervision should be incorporated in job descriptions.

7 **The content of supervision should be carefully defined, with boundaries agreed about what is and is not to be dealt with in supervision time. The processes to be used should also be made clear.**

Every supervisory relationship should be based on a clear understanding of the purpose and therefore the appropriate content of supervision.

At the start of a supervisory relationship, supervisor and supervisee should discuss and agree the likely content of their supervision sessions. This will involve mapping out general areas to be covered (eg review of recent practice, current problems and concerns, professional development and study/training needs), as well as identifying specific topics. Depending on the style of supervision, it may be helpful to make a long-term plan with agreed aims and objectives for a stated period or number of sessions.

Flexibility is important so that supervision can be used to respond to current needs and concerns, but some boundaries are needed to ensure that -

- supervision is used for the purposes agreed by the unit as a whole (see above)
- supervision is focused, purposeful and progressive
- demands upon the supervisor are held within appropriate limits
- the supervisee brings appropriate concerns to supervision and can expect those concerns to be dealt with.

The processes that will be used in supervision should also be discussed. It is important that both supervisor and supervisee understand the dynamics of their relationship so that they can find a way of working together effectively.

8 **The relationship between supervisor and supervisee should be formally constituted. Ground rules should be negotiated and agreed.**

In order to build the trust that is needed between supervisor and supervisee, it is vital that both partners understand the terms of their relationship. It is helpful if individual and mutual responsibilities are agreed at the start and expectations are recorded. These can be reviewed later. The supervisor should also make clear what skills, knowledge and experience he or she can (and cannot) bring to supervisory sessions.

Discussion of the terms of the supervisory relationship is especially important if the supervisor is also the supervisee's manager, since this can sometimes constrain the relationship.

Ground rules for the conduct of supervision should be negotiated at the beginning of any supervisory relationship and what is agreed should be recorded. Ground rules will cover, most importantly, confidentiality, and such issues as the exclusion of sexist, racist or otherwise insulting or offensive comment. It is vital that both supervisor and supervisee understand exactly what confidentiality means. Situations in which confidentiality would be broken should be clearly described.

The supervisee's right to change his or her supervisor should also be discussed. When clinical and managerial supervision are combined, supervisees may forego this right, but it is important that the implications and consequences of this are discussed.

Practical matters such as where to meet, how often, for how long, and arrangements for agenda-setting and note-taking also need to be agreed.

---

9 **It is essential that clinical supervision is monitored and evaluated. Supervisees and supervisors should play an equal part in these procedures.**

Methods for monitoring and evaluating the use of clinical supervision should be considered at planning stage.

A number of strategies will be needed in order to -

- assess the strengths and weaknesses of the system as a whole
- assess the strengths and weaknesses of supervision as experienced by individuals (both supervisors and supervisees)
- determine the future direction and development of supervision in the unit.

As the consumers of the service, it is particularly important that supervisees should be given opportunities to look objectively and critically at their experience of supervision. This should be done as a continuous process as well as by means of regular review; and both in conjunction with their supervisor and independently.

---

10 **Individual units need the support of their employing authority to implement and maintain a system of clinical supervision.**

For a unit to operate a successful system for clinical supervision, the practical commitment of staff within the unit should be matched by the political commitment of the trust or employing authority. It may otherwise be difficult for a unit to ensure that sufficient time is given to supervision within paid working hours and that training is provided to develop supervisory skills. The strategic implementation of clinical supervision, however, remains a matter for individual units.

Summary of the literature

Jean Faugier,
Senior Lecturer,
University of
Manchester

**Tony
Butterworth**,
Professor of
Community
Nursing,
University of
Manchester.

Clinical supervision, as a formal means of improving and monitoring practice, developed mainly in psychotherapy and counselling. It aims to improve skills, provide support and insights, and improve patient care by means of a formalised relationship or structure which involves regular interaction with a more skilled and experienced practitioner.

In nursing, clinical supervision has sometimes been viewed unsympathetically: "To many nurses, supervision means observation by an administrative superior who inspects, directs, controls and evaluates the nurse's work." (Platt-Koch, 1986)

If nursing is to move towards the implementation of clinical supervision as recommended in 'A Vision for the Future' (NHS ME, 1993), it is essential to examine the knowledge base available in the literature. This brief review offers some pointers to help the practitioner who recognises the need for information before action.

At first, the few examples of clinical supervision in nursing resulted from individual practitioners' dire needs and bitter experiences (Faugier, 1992). But it had almost always been viewed as the domain of specialist practitioners (Ivey, 1977), particularly in mental health nursing where recent moves towards individualised community care have made former group work models obsolete.

White (1990) and Ferguson (1992) emphasise that supervision is currently more developed among nurses working in community settings, especially in psychiatry, although Butterworth & Faugier (1993) point out that supervision relationships remain largely informal and ill-defined. However, when properly set up, Critchley (1987) notes that supervision does help nurses to observe, understand and describe more accurately, and to limit the impact of pre-conceptions about themselves and their clients. In a study

by Paunonen (1991) in Finland, nurses discovered a freedom and willingness to act.

The issue was further confused by the introduction of new terms such as 'mentor' and 'preceptor' from the USA (Collins & Scott, 1978). Darling (1984), a pioneer of mentorship in the USA, outlined the three characteristics of 'good mentors' as being an 'envisioner', a 'standard prodder' and a 'challenger'. Educationally, the advantages of mentorship are described by Puetz (1985) as enhancing students' skills and intellectual ability; Burnard (1989) sees those skills as transferrable to similar exchanges with patients, although Merriam (1983) and Fritsch & Strohlein (1988) emphasise the purely academic rather than practical nature of such skill acquisition. As for the concept of preceptorship, akin to that of probationary inspector, it is generally considered as positive in a number of (mainly American) studies: Clayton et al (1989), Pierce (1991), Myrick & Awrey (1988).

Apart from mental health nursing, where it has always had more reference to practice, clinical supervision when described in nursing tends to describe the educational aspects relating to mentorship and preceptorship (Twinn (1992), Pateman (1992). Hawkins & Shohet (1992) however stress its importance for self-awareness and on-going development, and as an essential guard against staleness, rigidity and defensiveness.

Houston (1990) and Simms (1993) want to get away from the literal meaning of supervision, arguing that its aim is to protect the client by developing the highest level of skill and professional attitudes within a trusting supportive relationship. This view is also expressed and expanded by Wright (1989).

Social work provides good lessons on the development of clinical supervision from an educative to a practical role. Middleman & Rhodes (1985) describe the evolution of this process towards an administrative, educative and supportive framework. In contrast, nursing has tended to rely more on 'hands-on' experience.

The 'continual learner' model of clinical supervision currently advocated in nursing (Butterworth & Faugier, 1992) is in line with the literature from psychotherapy (Wolberg, 1988 and Dryden, 1991), and counselling (Houston, 1990).

Wolberg (1988) and Dryden (1991) both emphasise the necessity for supervisors to fuse together the many disparate needs of supervisees, and to use, but not abuse, psychoanalytical theory.

Counselling, too, provides useful examples of supervision. Procter (1991) points out that it enables practitioners to "share working practice in detail" and "develop the ability to monitor one's own work."

Elsewhere, in psychotherapy and psychology, models have been developed in the USA by Stolenberg & Delworth (1987).

Models in clinical supervision

Procter (1986) suggests a model with three interactive functions termed as 'formative', 'restorative' and 'normative', which indicate the educational, supportive and managerial roles of the supervisor.

Faugier (1992) puts forward a 'growth and support' model, emphasising a number of important features in the supervisory relationship.

Frankham (1987) offers a model with twelve essential roles for the supervisor.

Hawkins & Shohet (1989) propose a 'two matrix' model based on common study of recorded material and the 'here and now' experience commonly used in counselling and psychotherapy.

Delivery models

Butterworth & Faugier (1992) suggest a number of practical options to organise supervision, while Hawkins & Shohet (1989) identify some common 'traps' to be avoided. Others, such as Ernst & Goodison (1981), Simms(1993) Munro et al (1979), and Douglas (1976), offer guidelines for setting up peer groups.

Supervision and clinical nursing leadership

Many writers have stressed the special developmental role of the 'clinical nurse specialist' for successful supervision: Ashworth (1975), Kerrane (1975), Wright (1986). Other authors have emphasised the relationship between reflective practice and supervision (Johns, 1993). The main emphasis in reflective practice is as Johns states "to give the practitioner access to a personal and practical knowledge in order to understand and respond therapeutically to the dynamics of caring." However there is a need to understand that reflection is a complex process which itself needs to be learned. If used inappropriately, it can leave the inexperienced practitioner 'reflecting' in a vacuum. Hence it is important to have in place the formalised structures of supervision which involve interaction with a practitioner whose knowledge base and skills are more highly developed than one's own. The capacity for spontaneous reflection on practice is a very high level skill which requires formalised supervision to aid its development as Casement (1985) points out. "During the course of being supervised, therapists [this can apply equally to nursing staff] need to acquire their own capacity for spontaneous reflection within the session. They can thus learn to watch themselves as well as the patient, now using the island of intellectual contemplation as the mental space within which the internal supervisor can begin to operate."

Training of clinical supervisors

Wright (1989) advocates the use of supervision seminars as instruments for training, while Clarkson & Gilbert (1991) suggest a much more structured approach through supervised practice with supervising clinicians remaining in the field. Claxton (1984) identifies potential obstacles ('beliefs') to good supervision training. Hawkins & Shohet (1989) put forward five types of training courses. Butterworth & Faugier (1992) propose a composite model of clinical supervision running through the whole professional life of nurses, from pre-registration to advanced practice.